CONTENTS

Happy Reading...

CHAPTER 1

INTRODUCTION

Weight loss is a journey embarked upon by individuals seeking to achieve a healthier body and lifestyle. It involves the intentional reduction of body weight, often with the goal of improving overall well-being, enhancing physical fitness, and reducing the risks of various health conditions. Weight loss can be achieved through a combination of balanced nutrition, regular physical activity, and sometimes medical interventions.

In recent times, the importance of weight loss has gained significant attention due to the rising prevalence of obesity and its associated health risks. Excess body weight can contribute to a range of health issues, including heart disease, diabetes, joint problems, and more. Therefore, pursuing weight loss is not just about appearance but also about taking proactive steps towards better health and quality of life.

It's important to approach weight loss with realistic expectations and a sustainable mindset. Crash diets and extreme measures are generally not recommended, as they can lead to nutrient deficiencies, muscle loss, and a cycle of weight regain. Instead, focusing on gradual, consistent changes to one's eating habits and physical activity level is often a more effective and lasting approach.

CHAPTER 2

UNDERSTANDING

WEIGHT LOSS

Understanding weight loss involves grasping the fundamental concepts and factors that contribute to the process of shedding excess body weight. Here are some key aspects to consider:

CALORIES IN VS. CALORIES OUT:

Weight loss is fundamentally driven by the balance between the number of calories you consume (calories in) and the number of calories you burn through various activities (calories out). When you consistently consume fewer calories than you expend, your body starts to use its stored fat for energy, leading to weight loss.

ENERGY BALANCE:

This concept ties into the calories in vs. calories out principle. Creating a calorie deficit by consuming fewer calories or increasing physical activity is essential for weight loss. Tracking your calorie intake and understanding the energy content of different foods can help you manage your energy balance effectively.

NUTRITION AND DIET:

The quality of the calories you consume matters. Opting for nutrient-dense foods, including vegetables, fruits, lean proteins, whole grains, and healthy fats, can support weight loss while providing essential nutrients for overall health.

METABOLISM:

Your metabolism influences how efficiently your body burns calories. Factors like age, genetics, muscle mass, and hormonal balance can impact your metabolic rate. Engaging in regular physical activity, particularly strength training, can help boost your metabolism.

PHYSICAL ACTIVITY:

Regular exercise not only burns calories but also improves your cardiovascular health, builds muscle, and supports overall well-being. Combining aerobic exercises (like walking, running, and cycling) with strength training can be effective for weight loss and body composition improvement.

BEHAVIORAL AND PSYCHOLOGICAL FACTORS:

Emotions, habits, stress, and social influences play a significant role in weight loss. Developing a positive relationship with food, managing stress, and addressing emotional triggers can help prevent overeating and promote long-term success.

SUSTAINABILITY:

Successful weight loss is often a gradual and sustainable process. Quick fixes or extreme diets tend to result in short-term results and can be difficult to maintain. Focus on making realistic and lasting lifestyle changes that you can incorporate into your daily routine.

HYDRATION AND SLEEP:

Drinking enough water and getting adequate sleep are important for weight loss. Proper hydration supports metabolism and appetite regulation, while quality sleep influences hormones that impact hunger and satiety.

MEDICAL CONSIDERATIONS:

If you have underlying health conditions or are considering significant weight loss, it's important to consult with a healthcare professional. They can provide personalized guidance, monitor your progress, and ensure your weight loss approach is safe and appropriate.

PLATEAUS AND SETBACKS:

Weight loss may not always follow a linear path. Plateaus and setbacks are normal and can be overcome with adjustments to your approach, such as modifying your diet or exercise routine.

In summary, understanding weight loss involves recognizing the interplay between calories, nutrition, physical activity, metabolism, psychological factors, and overall health. A well-rounded approach that addresses these factors is key to achieving and maintaining successful and sustainable weight loss.

CHAPTER 3
HEALTHY EATING HABITS

Healthy eating habits play a crucial role in weight loss and overall well-being. Here are some tips to help you develop and maintain a balanced and effective approach to healthy eating for weight loss:

EAT WHOLE, NUTRIENT-DENSE FOODS:

Focus on consuming whole foods that are rich in nutrients and low in empty calories. These include vegetables, fruits, lean proteins, whole grains, nuts, seeds, and legumes.

CONTROL PORTION SIZES:

Pay attention to portion sizes to avoid overeating. Use smaller plates and bowls, and be mindful of portion sizes when eating out.

STAY HYDRATED:

Drink plenty of water throughout the day. Sometimes, our bodies confuse thirst with hunger, leading to unnecessary snacking.

BALANCED MEALS:

Aim for balanced meals that include a combination of protein, healthy fats, fiber, and carbohydrates. This can help stabilize blood sugar levels and keep you feeling full and satisfied.

LIMIT PROCESSED FOODS:

Minimize or eliminate processed and refined foods, such as sugary snacks, fast food, and sugary beverages. These foods often contain empty calories and lack essential nutrients.

COOK AT HOME:

Cooking your own meals gives you more control over ingredients and cooking methods. It also helps you make healthier choices.

MINDFUL EATING:

Pay attention to your body's hunger and fullness cues. Eat slowly, savoring each bite, and stop when you feel comfortably satisfied.

FIBER-RICH FOODS:

Include plenty of high-fiber foods in your diet, such as whole grains, vegetables, fruits, and legumes. Fiber helps you feel full and aids in digestion.

HEALTHY SNACKING:

Choose nutritious snacks like yogurt, fruits, nuts, and vegetables. Avoid mindless snacking and opt for portion-controlled options.

REGULAR MEALS:

Don't skip meals, especially breakfast. Eating regular meals can help prevent overeating later in the day.

LIMIT ADDED SUGAR:

Reduce your intake of added sugars found in sugary snacks, desserts, and sweetened beverages. Read labels to identify hidden sources of sugar.

INCLUDE LEAN PROTEINS:

Protein helps you feel full and supports muscle growth. Include lean sources such as poultry, fish, tofu, legumes, and low-fat dairy.

HEALTHY FATS:

Incorporate sources of healthy fats, such as avocados, nuts, seeds, and olive oil. These fats are essential for various bodily functions.

PLAN AHEAD:

Plan your meals and snacks in advance to avoid impulsive, unhealthy choices when hungry.

REGULAR EXERCISE:

Combine healthy eating habits with regular physical activity to enhance weight loss and overall health.

GET ADEQUATE SLEEP:

Aim for 7-9 hours of quality sleep each night, as lack of sleep can affect hormones related to hunger and appetite.

MANAGE STRESS:

Practice stress-reduction techniques like meditation, deep breathing, or yoga. Stress can lead to emotional eating and weight gain.

Remember that weight loss is a gradual process, and it's important to focus on making sustainable lifestyle changes rather than pursuing quick fixes. Consult a healthcare professional or registered dietitian before making significant changes to your diet or exercise routine, especially if you have any underlying health conditions.

CHAPTER 4

MEAL PLANNING

AND

PREPARATION

Effective meal planning and preparation are essential components of a successful weight loss journey. Here's a step-by-step guide to help you plan and prepare meals that support your weight loss goals:

SET CLEAR GOALS:

Define your weight loss goals and understand your daily calorie and nutrient needs. This information will guide your meal planning.

CREATE A MEAL PLAN:

Design a weekly meal plan that includes breakfast, lunch, dinner, and snacks. Focus on nutrient-dense foods and balanced meals.

CHOOSE WHOLE FOODS:

Select whole, unprocessed foods like lean proteins, vegetables, fruits, whole grains, nuts, seeds, and legumes. These foods are rich in nutrients and fiber, which aid in satiety.

PORTION CONTROL:

Pay attention to portion sizes to avoid overeating. Use measuring cups, a kitchen scale, or visual cues to help you estimate appropriate portions.

PREP AHEAD:

Set aside time each week for meal preparation. Prepare larger batches of staple ingredients like cooked grains, lean proteins, and chopped vegetables to use throughout the week.

PLAN BALANCED MEALS:

Ensure each meal contains a source of lean protein, healthy fats, and fiber-rich carbohydrates. This combination helps keep you full and satisfied.

SNACK WISELY:

Have healthy snacks on hand, like cut-up veggies, fruits, yogurt, or nuts, to prevent unhealthy choices when hunger strikes.

USE COOKING METHODS WISELY:

Opt for cooking methods that use minimal added fats, such as baking, grilling, steaming, and sautéing with small amounts of olive oil.

MINDFUL EATING:

Sit down and eat your meals mindfully, savoring each bite. Avoid distractions like screens or work while eating.

PRE-PORTION MEALS:

Divide prepared foods into portion-sized containers. This helps with portion control and makes grabbing a meal or snack convenient.

KEEP HEALTHY STAPLES:

Maintain a well-stocked pantry with items like whole grains, canned beans, canned tuna, nuts, seeds, and healthy cooking oils.

PLAN FOR TREATS:

Allow yourself occasional treats to prevent feelings of deprivation. Plan these treats into your weekly meal plan in moderation.

STAY HYDRATED:

Drink water throughout the day. Sometimes, our bodies confuse thirst with hunger.

ADJUST AS NEEDED:

Monitor your progress and adjust your meal plan as necessary. Listen to your body's cues and make modifications based on how you feel.

SEEK PROFESSIONAL GUIDANCE:

Consult a registered dietitian or nutritionist for personalized meal planning advice tailored to your needs and preferences.

SAMPLE DAY OF MEALS:

Breakfast: Scrambled eggs with spinach and tomatoes, whole-grain toast, and a side of berries.

Lunch: Grilled chicken salad with mixed greens, cucumbers, bell peppers, and a light vinaigrette dressing.

Snack: Greek yogurt with a sprinkle of nuts and a small apple.

Dinner: Baked salmon with quinoa and steamed broccoli.

Snack: Carrot sticks with hummus.

Remember that meal planning and preparation require consistency and patience. Gradually incorporate these practices into your routine, and make adjustments based on what works best for you. The key is to create a sustainable plan that supports your weight loss goals while also promoting overall health and well-being.

CHAPTER 5

EXERCISE AND PHYSICAL ACTIVITY

Exercise and physical activity are important components of a successful weight loss journey. When combined with a healthy diet, they can help you achieve your weight loss goals and improve your overall fitness and well-being. Here's a guide to incorporating exercise and physical activity into your weight loss plan:

CHOOSE ACTIVITIES YOU ENJOY:

Engage in physical activities you genuinely enjoy, as you're more likely to stick with them. Whether it's walking, cycling, swimming, dancing, or playing a sport, find activities that make you feel motivated and excited.

START SLOWLY:

If you're new to exercise, start with low-impact activities and gradually increase the intensity and duration. This helps prevent injury and allows your body to adapt over time.

MIX CARDIOVASCULAR AND STRENGTH TRAINING:

Incorporate both cardiovascular exercises (like walking, jogging, cycling, or swimming) and strength training (using weights, resistance bands, or bodyweight exercises). Cardio burns calories and improves cardiovascular health, while strength training builds lean muscle mass, which boosts metabolism.

AIM FOR REGULARITY:

Strive for at least 150 minutes of moderate-intensity or 75 minutes of vigorous-intensity aerobic activity per week, along with two days of strength training. You can break these sessions into smaller chunks throughout the week.

HIGH-INTENSITY INTERVAL TRAINING (HIIT):

Consider incorporating HIIT workouts, which alternate between short bursts of intense activity and periods of rest. HIIT can be effective for burning calories and improving cardiovascular fitness in a shorter amount of time.

INCLUDE FLEXIBILITY AND BALANCE EXERCISES:

Incorporate activities like yoga, Pilates, or stretching to improve flexibility and balance. These exercises also promote relaxation and reduce stress.

SET REALISTIC GOALS:

Set achievable fitness goals that are specific, measurable, and time-bound. Tracking your progress can help keep you motivated and focused.

STAY CONSISTENT:

Consistency is key to seeing results. Make exercise a regular part of your routine and prioritize it just like any other important activity.

LISTEN TO YOUR BODY:

Pay attention to how your body feels during and after exercise. Rest when needed and avoid pushing yourself too hard, especially when starting out.

STAY HYDRATED:

Drink water before, during, and after exercise to stay hydrated and support your body's performance.

WARM-UP AND COOL DOWN:

Always start with a proper warm-up and end with a cool-down to prevent injury and improve flexibility.

MONITOR PROGRESS:

Track your workouts, noting the exercises, duration, and intensity. Seeing your progress can be motivating and help you adjust your routine as needed.

CONSULT A PROFESSIONAL:

If you have any health concerns or medical conditions, consult a healthcare professional before starting a new exercise program. A fitness trainer or coach can also provide guidance on proper form and techniques.

STAY POSITIVE AND PATIENT:

Remember that weight loss takes time. Focus on the positive changes exercise brings to your overall health and well-being, and celebrate your achievements along the way.

Combining a balanced diet with regular exercise and physical activity can lead to sustainable weight loss and improved fitness. It's important to find an approach that works for you and fits into your lifestyle, so you can create healthy habits that you can maintain over the long term.

CHAPTER 6

LIFESTYLE CHANGES FOR SUCCESS

Achieving successful and sustainable weight loss requires making meaningful lifestyle changes. Here are some key lifestyle adjustments that can contribute to your weight loss journey:

SET REALISTIC GOALS:

Set achievable and specific weight loss goals. Focus on gradual progress rather than rapid changes.

MINDFUL EATING:

Practice mindful eating by paying attention to hunger and fullness cues. Eat slowly and savour each bite to prevent overeating.

PORTION CONTROL:

Learn to recognize appropriate portion sizes and avoid oversized portions. Use smaller plates and bowls to help with portion control.

REGULAR PHYSICAL ACTIVITY:

Incorporate regular exercise into your routine. Aim for a combination of cardiovascular exercises, strength training, and flexibility activities.

SLEEP QUALITY:

Prioritize getting enough quality sleep each night. Lack of sleep can disrupt hormones that regulate appetite and lead to weight gain.

STRESS MANAGEMENT:

Implement stress-reduction techniques such as meditation, deep breathing, yoga, or spending time in nature. Stress can contribute to emotional eating and weight gain.

BALANCED DIET:

Focus on a balanced diet rich in whole, nutrient-dense foods. Include a variety of vegetables, fruits, lean proteins, whole grains, and healthy fats.

HYDRATION:

Drink plenty of water throughout the day. Water helps control appetite and supports metabolism.

MEAL PLANNING:

Plan and prepare meals ahead of time to avoid last-minute unhealthy choices. This can help you stick to your dietary goals.

LIMIT PROCESSED FOODS:

Minimize or eliminate processed and sugary foods, as they often contain empty calories and lack essential nutrients.

SUPPORTIVE ENVIRONMENT:

Surround yourself with people who support your weight loss journey. Communicate your goals to friends and family so they can provide encouragement.

ACCOUNTABILITY:

Consider joining a weight loss group, partnering with a friend, or hiring a coach to provide accountability and motivation.

MONITOR PROGRESS:

Track your food intake, exercise routines, and progress over time. This can help you identify patterns and make necessary adjustments.

BE KIND TO YOURSELF:

Embrace self-compassion and avoid being too hard on yourself. Weight loss is a journey with ups and downs; celebrate your successes and learn from setbacks.

AVOID EXTREME DIETS:

Avoid crash diets or extreme restrictions. Focus on sustainable changes that you can maintain in the long term.

GRADUAL CHANGES:

Make gradual lifestyle changes to avoid feeling overwhelmed. Small, consistent adjustments can lead to lasting results.

CELEBRATE NON-SCALE VICTORIES:

Celebrate achievements beyond the scale, such as increased energy, improved fitness, better sleep, and enhanced mood.

PROFESSIONAL GUIDANCE:

Consult a registered dietitian or healthcare professional for personalized guidance and support throughout your weight loss journey.

Remember that every individual's weight loss journey is unique. It's important to find an approach that aligns with your preferences, needs, and circumstances. Making these lifestyle changes can not only help you lose weight but also improve your overall health and well-being.

CHAPTER 7
TRACKING AND MONITORING PROGRESS

Tracking and monitoring your progress is essential for staying on track with your weight loss goals and making necessary adjustments. Here's how you can effectively track and monitor your progress:

KEEP A FOOD JOURNAL:

Record what you eat and drink each day. Be detailed and include portion sizes. This helps you become more aware of your eating habits and identify areas for improvement.

USE A TRACKING APP:

There are numerous mobile apps that can help you track your daily food intake, exercise, and even monitor your nutrient intake. Examples include MyFitnessPal, Lose It!, and Cronometer.

TAKE BEFORE AND AFTER PHOTOS:

Capture photos of yourself at the start of your weight loss journey and periodically throughout. Visual changes can be motivating, especially when the scale might not reflect immediate progress.

WEIGH YOURSELF REGULARLY:

Weigh yourself at the same time of day and under the same conditions (e.g., in the morning after using the bathroom). Keep in mind that weight can fluctuate daily due to factors like hydration and hormones.

MEASURE BODY CIRCUMFERENCES:

Use a tape measure to track changes in your waist, hips, arms, and legs. This can provide a more accurate picture of your progress than weight alone.

MONITOR FITNESS AND STRENGTH:

Track improvements in your fitness levels, such as increased stamina, higher weights lifted, or longer distances walked or run.

KEEP A WORKOUT LOG:

Document your workouts, including exercises, sets, reps, and weights used. This helps you see progress over time and adjust your routines as needed.

SET NON-SCALE GOALS:

Focus on non-scale victories, such as better sleep, improved energy, increased flexibility, or reduced cravings.

TRACK MOOD AND ENERGY LEVELS:

Note how you feel physically and emotionally throughout the day. This can help you identify patterns between your behaviors and how you feel.

EVALUATE PORTION CONTROL:

Check in regularly to ensure you're maintaining appropriate portion sizes and not slipping into overeating.

REFLECT ON CHALLENGES AND SUCCESSES:

Take time to reflect on your successes and challenges. What strategies are working well, and where do you need to make adjustments?

ADJUST YOUR APPROACH:

Use your tracking data to make informed decisions about your diet and exercise. If progress is stalling, consider modifying your routine or seeking professional guidance.

BE PATIENT AND REALISTIC:

Remember that progress might not always be linear. Weight loss can vary from week to week, but the overall trend is what matters.

CELEBRATE MILESTONES:

Reward yourself when you achieve specific milestones. Treat yourself to something non-food-related that brings you joy.

CONSULT A PROFESSIONAL:

If you're unsure how to interpret your progress or need guidance, consider working with a registered dietitian, personal trainer, or healthcare professional.

Consistency is key when it comes to tracking and monitoring progress. Regularly reviewing your data and making adjustments based on your findings can help you stay motivated and stay on the path toward reaching your weight loss goals.

CHAPTER 8
OVERCOMING
CHALLENGES

Weight loss can be a challenging journey, but with the right strategies and mindset, you can overcome obstacles and achieve your goals. Here are some common challenges people face during weight loss and how to overcome them:

LACK OF MOTIVATION:

Solution: Find your "why" – identify your reasons for wanting to lose weight. Set realistic goals and remind yourself of the benefits you'll gain from achieving them.

EMOTIONAL EATING:

Solution: Practice mindfulness and develop alternative coping mechanisms for stress, boredom, or other emotions. Engage in activities you enjoy or seek support from friends, family, or a therapist.

PLATEAUS:

Solution: Plateaus are normal. Focus on non-scale victories, reassess your goals, adjust your diet or exercise routine, and remind yourself of how far you've come.

CRAVINGS:

Solution: Allow yourself occasional treats in moderation, plan satisfying and nutritious meals, stay hydrated, and keep healthy snacks on hand.

SOCIAL PRESSURE AND TEMPTATIONS:

Solution: Communicate your goals with friends and family, choose healthier options at social gatherings, and practice assertiveness in declining unhealthy foods.

TIME CONSTRAINTS:

Solution: Prioritize meal planning, preparation, and exercise. Incorporate short bursts of activity throughout the day, and choose efficient workouts like high-intensity interval training (HIIT).

INCONSISTENT RESULTS:

Solution: Focus on long-term trends rather than daily fluctuations. Stay patient and stay consistent with healthy habits.

NEGATIVE SELF-TALK:

Solution: Practice self-compassion and positive self-talk. Replace negative thoughts with encouraging and affirming statements.

LACK OF SUPPORT:

Solution: Seek support from friends, family, or a support group. Consider joining online communities or finding a weight loss buddy.

FEAR OF FAILURE:

Solution: Embrace failures as learning opportunities. Shift your mindset to view setbacks as part of the journey and keep moving forward.

UNREALISTIC EXPECTATIONS:

Solution: Set achievable, incremental goals. Focus on sustainable changes and long-term health, rather than quick fixes.

PHYSICAL LIMITATIONS OR HEALTH CONDITIONS:

Solution: Consult a healthcare professional before starting any weight loss program. They can help you design a safe and effective plan tailored to your individual needs.

BOREDOM OR MONOTONY:

Solution: Keep your workouts and meals varied and interesting. Try new recipes, exercise routines, or activities to keep things fresh.

ALL-OR-NOTHING MENTALITY:

Solution: Avoid perfectionism. Focus on progress, not perfection, and don't let minor slip-ups derail your entire effort.

COMPARISONS TO OTHERS:

Solution: Focus on your own progress and journey. Remember that everyone's body is unique and progresses at its own pace.

Remember that weight loss is a gradual process, and setbacks are a normal part of the journey. The key is to stay committed, resilient, and adaptable. Celebrate your successes, no matter how small, and keep your focus on the positive changes you're making for your health and well-being.

CHAPTER 9

MAINTAINING

WEIGHT LOSS

Maintaining weight loss is often as challenging as achieving it in the first place. However, with the right strategies and mindset, you can increase your chances of successfully keeping the weight off over the long term. Here are some tips for maintaining weight loss:

MINDFUL EATING:

Continue practicing mindful eating even after reaching your goal weight. Pay attention to hunger and fullness cues, savour your meals, and avoid eating out of boredom or emotions.

REGULAR PHYSICAL ACTIVITY:

Keep up with your exercise routine. Aim for a mix of cardiovascular exercises, strength training, and flexibility activities to maintain your fitness level and metabolism.

SET REALISTIC GOALS:

Shift your focus from weight loss to weight maintenance. Set new goals related to maintaining your current weight and overall well-being.

MONITOR YOUR PROGRESS:

Continue tracking your food intake, exercise, and progress. Regular monitoring can help you catch any gradual weight changes and make necessary adjustments.

STAY HYDRATED:

Drink plenty of water throughout the day. Proper hydration supports metabolism and helps control appetite.

STAY ACTIVE:

Incorporate physical activity into your daily life, such as walking, taking the stairs, or participating in active hobbies you enjoy.

PLAN MEALS AND SNACKS:

Continue meal planning and preparation to ensure you're making balanced and nutritious choices.

MANAGE STRESS:

Practice stress management techniques like meditation, deep breathing, or yoga to prevent emotional eating.

CELEBRATE NON-SCALE VICTORIES:

Focus on achievements beyond the scale, such as improved energy, fitness levels, and overall health.

KEEP LEARNING:

Stay informed about nutrition, fitness, and healthy habits. Knowledge empowers you to make informed choices.

AVOID EXTREMES:

Steer clear of extreme diets or overly restrictive eating patterns. Aim for a sustainable approach that you can maintain in the long term.

SOCIAL SUPPORT:

Continue seeking support from friends, family, or support groups. Share your goals and challenges to stay accountable.

REGULAR CHECK-INS:

Schedule periodic check-ins with a healthcare professional or registered dietitian to assess your progress and make any necessary adjustments.

FLEXIBILITY:

Embrace flexibility in your eating and exercise routine. Life will have its ups and downs, and adapting to change is key to long-term success.

PRACTICE SELF-COMPASSION:

Be kind to yourself and avoid self-criticism. Remember that weight maintenance is a lifelong journey with occasional fluctuations.

CELEBRATE WITHOUT FOOD:

Find ways to celebrate achievements or milestones that don't involve food. Treat yourself to non-food rewards like a spa day, new clothing, or a hobby you enjoy.

STAY POSITIVE:

Cultivate a positive attitude and believe in your ability to maintain your weight loss. Surround yourself with positivity and people who support your goals.

Remember that maintaining weight loss is an ongoing commitment to a healthy lifestyle. Stay patient, adaptable, and focused on the habits that helped you lose weight in the first place. By making healthy choices a permanent part of your life, you can enjoy the benefits of your hard work and dedication.

CHAPTER 10
CONCLUSION

In conclusion, embarking on a weight loss journey requires a multifaceted approach that encompasses healthy eating habits, regular physical activity, and a supportive mindset. While weight loss can be challenging, it is achievable through consistent effort and dedication to making sustainable lifestyle changes.

Starting with a well-balanced and nutrient-dense diet lays the foundation for successful weight loss. Prioritizing whole foods, controlling portion sizes, and being mindful of eating habits contribute to creating a healthier relationship with food.

Complementing your dietary changes with regular physical activity is essential for both shedding excess pounds and maintaining overall well-being. A combination of cardiovascular exercises, strength training, and flexibility routines not only helps burn calories but also improves fitness levels and boosts metabolism.

The journey of weight loss is not without its hurdles. Overcoming challenges like emotional eating, plateaus, and maintaining motivation requires resilience, patience, and a positive attitude. Monitoring progress, setting realistic goals, seeking support from professionals or peers, and practicing self-compassion can all contribute to overcoming obstacles along the way.

As you work towards your weight loss goals, remember that your ultimate aim is not just a number on the scale, but rather improved health, increased energy, enhanced self-confidence, and an overall better quality of life. Embracing a holistic approach to weight loss that considers both physical and mental well-being will set you on a path towards long-term success and a healthier, happier you.

In the journey of weight loss, the path is often challenging and requires dedication, perseverance, and a strong commitment to one's goals. It's a process that extends far beyond just shedding pounds; it's about embracing a healthier lifestyle, both physically and mentally. As the scale shows progress, so does the growth in self-confidence, energy levels, and overall well-being.

Remember that weight loss is not a one-size-fits-all endeavour. Each individual's experience is unique, and there's no "quick fix" solution. It's essential to approach weight loss with a balanced perspective, focusing on sustainable changes that promote long-term health rather than temporary results.

The End

9 798822 310609